# Exocrine Pancreatic Insufficiency (EPI) Cookbook

## Easy, Gut-Friendly Recipes for Managing EPI Symptoms, Boosting Digestion, and Supporting Pancreatic Health

# Nelson zavian

# DISCLIAMER

The information contained in this book, *Exocrine Pancreatic Insufficiency (EPI) Cookbook*, is intended for educational and informational purposes only. It is not a substitute for professional medical advice, diagnosis, or treatment. Always seek the advice of your physician or other qualified health provider with any questions you may have regarding a medical condition or dietary concerns. Never disregard professional medical advice or delay in seeking it because of something you have read in this book.

While the recipes and dietary guidelines provided are designed to support individuals managing Exocrine Pancreatic Insufficiency (EPI), individual nutritional needs may vary. It is important to consult with a healthcare provider or registered dietitian before making significant changes to your diet, especially if you have underlying health conditions or are taking medications. The author and publisher of this book are not responsible for any adverse effects or consequences resulting from the use or application of the information contained herein.

This book may reference or mention various individuals, products, websites, organizations, or other names. Such references are intended solely for informational purposes and do not constitute an endorsement of any specific individual, product, or organization.

By reading this book, you acknowledge and accept that you are responsible for your own health and well-being. The author and publisher will not be held liable for any direct, indirect, incidental, or consequential damages arising from the use or misuse of the information provided in this book. Always prioritize your health and consult with qualified professionals as needed.

# ABOUT THIS BOOK

The "Exocrine Pancreatic Insufficiency (EPI) Cookbook" serves as a vital resource for individuals navigating the complexities of managing EPI through diet. Exocrine pancreatic insufficiency is a condition where the pancreas does not produce enough digestive enzymes, leading to difficulties in digesting food properly. This cookbook provides not only a comprehensive understanding of EPI but also emphasizes the importance of a gut-friendly diet that can significantly alleviate symptoms and enhance overall health. The knowledge presented within its pages empowers readers to take control of their dietary choices, ultimately leading to improved digestive health and quality of life.

Understanding the relationship between diet and pancreatic health is crucial for those with EPI. The book meticulously outlines how specific foods can impact digestion and overall well-being, guiding readers through the essentials of nutrient management. By incorporating easy-to-digest ingredients and emphasizing a balanced intake of macronutrients—carbohydrates, proteins, and fats—the cookbook equips individuals with the tools needed to alleviate symptoms and promote better digestion. This nutritional guidance helps demystify dietary restrictions and empowers readers to embrace food as a source of nourishment rather than a source of anxiety.

A standout feature of this cookbook is its structured approach to recipes, categorized to meet various dietary needs. Each recipe is crafted with care, ensuring that they are not only nutritious but also palatable. By offering a diverse array of meal options—ranging from appetizers to desserts—the book caters to different tastes while prioritizing gut health. The focus on low-FODMAP and easily digestible recipes means that individuals can enjoy meals that are both satisfying and safe, making it easier to incorporate healthy eating into daily life.

Moreover, the "Exocrine Pancreatic Insufficiency (EPI) Cookbook" goes beyond just recipes; it fosters a sense of community and support through shared success stories. These testimonials not only inspire hope but also demonstrate the practical effectiveness of dietary changes. Readers will find encouragement in the experiences of others who have successfully managed EPI symptoms through dedicated dietary adjustments, reinforcing the notion that they are not alone in their journey.

The inclusion of comprehensive sections on grocery shopping and meal preparation further enriches the reader's experience. By providing insights on how to select gut-friendly foods and the best cooking techniques for EPI management, the book becomes an essential companion in the kitchen. It demystifies the grocery shopping process, ensuring that individuals feel confident in their ability to curate meals that promote pancreatic health and digestion. The practical advice is not only empowering but also fosters a proactive approach to health management.

In addition to addressing immediate dietary needs, this cookbook lays the groundwork for long-term health and wellness. By equipping readers with the knowledge of essential nutrients, hydration, and cooking methods tailored to their needs, it encourages a lifestyle that prioritizes digestive health. This commitment to holistic well-being is reflected throughout the book, making it an indispensable tool for anyone seeking to improve their quality of life while managing the challenges of exocrine pancreatic insufficiency. Through its blend of informative content and accessible recipes, this cookbook truly stands out as a beacon of hope and guidance for those on the path to better health.

# Table of Contents

# Introduction

## Understanding Exocrine Pancreatic Insufficiency (EPI)

Exocrine Pancreatic Insufficiency (EPI) is a condition where the pancreas doesn't produce enough digestive enzymes, leading to difficulty in breaking down and absorbing nutrients. Common symptoms include bloating, diarrhea, and weight loss, as food passes through the digestive system without being properly broken down. EPI can occur as a result of chronic pancreatitis, cystic fibrosis, or other pancreatic disorders.

Managing EPI requires enzyme replacement therapy and a carefully planned diet. By including easily digestible foods, low in fat and fiber, individuals can support digestion while minimizing symptoms. Enzyme supplements taken with meals help break down food, and combining this approach with gut-friendly, nutrient-dense foods can improve both symptom management and overall health.

## Importance of a Gut-Friendly Diet

A gut-friendly diet for individuals with EPI focuses on foods that are easy to digest and supportive of enzyme function. This often includes lean proteins, low-fat dairy, fruits without seeds or peels, and cooked vegetables. Foods high in fat, fiber, and sugar should be limited, as they can aggravate symptoms like bloating and gas.

Incorporating foods that are rich in probiotics, such as yogurt or kefir, helps maintain a healthy balance of gut bacteria, aiding digestion. Additionally, eating small, frequent meals allows the digestive system to process food more efficiently and reduces strain on the pancreas. A well-balanced diet, combined with enzyme supplements, promotes better nutrient absorption and helps prevent malnutrition.

## How Proper Nutrition Affects Pancreatic Health

Proper nutrition plays a vital role in managing EPI and supporting pancreatic health. When the pancreas is unable to produce enough enzymes, the body struggles to break down fats, proteins, and carbohydrates. To ease this burden, a diet that reduces pancreatic workload is essential. Low-fat foods, such as lean meats, fish, and egg whites, are easier for the body to process and reduce strain on the pancreas.

Including nutrient-dense foods like avocados, nuts, and leafy greens ensures the body receives essential vitamins and minerals despite digestive challenges. Hydration is also key; drinking plenty of water helps with digestion and prevents dehydration from symptoms like diarrhea. With the right nutritional approach, EPI patients can maintain their health and reduce complications.

## Key Principles for Managing EPI Symptoms

Managing EPI symptoms effectively requires adherence to key dietary principles, starting with enzyme supplementation. Pancreatic enzyme replacement therapy (PERT) should be taken with every meal to ensure that fats, proteins, and carbohydrates are properly digested. Without these enzymes, nutrients may pass through the digestive system undigested, causing malabsorption and gastrointestinal discomfort.

Additionally, portion control is crucial. Small, frequent meals are easier to digest and allow for better enzyme function. Pairing low-fat foods with complex carbohydrates, such as whole grains and vegetables, stabilizes blood sugar levels and promotes better digestion. Avoiding high-fat and high-fiber foods can significantly reduce bloating, gas, and discomfort.

## Overview of Recipe Categories

The recipe categories in this cookbook are specifically tailored to EPI-friendly meals that promote digestion and pancreatic health. Categories include breakfast, lunch, dinner, snacks, and beverages. For breakfast, recipes may feature low-fat, protein-rich options like egg-white omelets or smoothies with enzyme supplements added for easier digestion.

Lunch and dinner focus on lean proteins like chicken, fish, and plant-based alternatives, paired with simple carbohydrates such as quinoa or sweet potatoes. Snacks are light and nutritious, including options like yogurt with fruit or boiled eggs. Beverages, including herbal teas and enzyme-boosted smoothies, aid digestion and provide hydration without overloading the digestive system. Each category prioritizes easy-to-digest ingredients that support symptom management.

# The Importance of This Diet Cookbook

**Managing EPI Symptoms:** This cookbook is designed specifically for individuals with Exocrine Pancreatic Insufficiency (EPI), offering recipes that are easy on the digestive system. EPI sufferers often struggle with nutrient absorption due to insufficient pancreatic enzymes. By following these gut-friendly recipes, you can reduce symptoms like bloating, gas, and diarrhea, and ensure you're getting the right balance of nutrients. Each recipe is crafted to be low in fat and high in easily digestible proteins and carbohydrates, which helps in alleviating the strain on the digestive system.

**Supporting Pancreatic Health:** The cookbook emphasizes ingredients that support pancreatic health, such as lean proteins, whole grains, and fruits. By focusing on foods that are gentle on the pancreas, it helps maintain a balanced digestive process. For example, recipes include options like steamed fish and quinoa, which are both nutrient-dense and easy to digest. Incorporating these foods into your diet can help your pancreas function more effectively and promote overall digestive wellness.

# How This Book Can Help You Achieve a Better Life

**Boosting Digestion:** This book provides practical recipes that enhance digestion and nutrient absorption. Each dish is designed to be low in irritating substances and high in essential nutrients. For instance, a simple recipe for chicken and vegetable soup offers a balanced, easy-to-digest meal that supports digestion and helps manage EPI symptoms. By following the meal plans and recipes, you'll likely notice improvements in digestive comfort and overall well-being.

**Enhancing Daily Living:** Adopting the recipes from this cookbook can significantly improve your daily quality of life. By focusing on meals that are tailored for EPI management, you reduce the discomfort associated with poor digestion and nutrient malabsorption. For example, the cookbook includes quick, nutritious meals like a lentil and spinach salad that are not only gut-friendly but also convenient for busy lifestyles. This approach makes it easier to maintain a healthy diet while managing EPI effectively.

# Success stories

## Sarah's Journey to Wellness

Sarah, a 38-year-old teacher, struggled with severe digestive issues and weight loss due to EPI. Despite trying various treatments and diets, she found little relief until she discovered your cookbook. The easy-to-follow recipes allowed her to prepare gut-friendly meals that were both nutritious and tailored to her condition. Within weeks of following the cookbook, Sarah experienced significant improvements in digestion, energy levels, and overall well-being. The cookbook's emphasis on balancing nutrients and incorporating digestive aids helped her regain her health and confidence. Sarah now shares her success story with others in her EPI support group, recommending your book as a crucial resource for managing their symptoms.

## John's Transformation

John, a 45-year-old IT consultant, had been diagnosed with EPI for several years and felt overwhelmed by the dietary restrictions imposed by his condition. After purchasing your cookbook, John found that the simple, yet effective recipes made meal planning and preparation much easier. He appreciated the book's focus on gut-friendly ingredients and practical cooking tips. As he incorporated these recipes into his daily routine, he noticed a dramatic improvement in his digestive health and a reduction in EPI-related symptoms. John credits the cookbook with helping him achieve better digestive comfort and a more balanced lifestyle, leading to increased productivity and a more enjoyable life.

## Emily's Health Revival

Emily, a 29-year-old graphic designer, was diagnosed with EPI after struggling with chronic abdominal pain and malnutrition. She began using your cookbook as a guide to adapt her diet to her new needs. The cookbook's emphasis on easy-to-prepare meals that are both nutritious and tailored to EPI management made a significant difference in her health. Emily found relief from her symptoms and was able to enjoy a wider variety of foods without discomfort. Her overall health improved, including her energy levels and mental clarity. Emily now uses your cookbook as a reference and often recommends it to others facing similar challenges, praising its role in her journey to better health.

## Michael's Dietary Revolution

Michael, a 52-year-old retired firefighter, had struggled with EPI-related complications for years, leading to frequent hospital visits and dietary confusion. After discovering your cookbook, he was thrilled by the straightforward approach and practical recipes it offered. By following the cookbook's guidelines, Michael experienced a noticeable improvement in his digestion and a reduction in EPI symptoms. He found that the recipes were not only beneficial but also enjoyable to make and eat. Michael's health transformation led him to become an advocate for the cookbook within his community, highlighting how it facilitated a positive change in his life and significantly improved his quality of life.

# Chapter 1:

# What a Healthy Diet Must Include

## Essential Nutrients for EPI Management

Managing Exocrine Pancreatic Insufficiency (EPI) requires focusing on specific nutrients that support digestion and overall gut health. The body lacks the enzymes to break down food effectively, so it's important to choose nutrient-rich, easily digestible foods. Focus on lean proteins like fish and chicken, along with healthy fats such as olive oil and avocado. These options are easier on the pancreas and help to ensure you're getting the calories and nutrients needed without overwhelming the digestive system.

In addition to proteins and fats, carbohydrates play a key role, but it's crucial to select easily digestible carbs like rice, oats, and sweet potatoes. Avoid processed foods and opt for natural, whole grains that provide sustained energy. Incorporating digestive enzymes with meals can further help in breaking down these nutrients, aiding absorption and reducing symptoms like bloating and discomfort.

## Balancing Macronutrients: Carbohydrates, Proteins, and Fats

Balancing macronutrients is vital for EPI management as the pancreas struggles to produce enzymes that break down food. For carbohydrates, opt for easily digestible, low-fiber options like white rice, potatoes, and well-cooked vegetables, which put less strain on your digestive system.

Whole grains and raw vegetables, though healthy, may be more difficult to digest without enzyme supplementation, so always pair them with pancreatic enzyme replacement therapy (PERT).

When it comes to proteins, stick to lean sources such as chicken, turkey, fish, or plant-based options like tofu. For fats, prioritize healthy fats from avocados, nuts, seeds, and olive oil, while avoiding high-fat meals that can trigger EPI symptoms. Always use PERT when eating fats, as they are the most challenging macronutrient for those with EPI to digest.

## Importance of Fiber in Digestion

Fiber plays a crucial role in gut health, but those with EPI must be cautious. Soluble fiber, found in foods like oats, apples, and carrots, is easier on the digestive system and can help regulate bowel movements. This type of fiber dissolves in water and forms a gel-like substance that aids digestion without irritating the gut.

In contrast, insoluble fiber, found in whole grains and raw vegetables, may cause discomfort and exacerbate symptoms in those with EPI. It's important to gradually introduce fiber into the diet while ensuring proper enzyme supplementation to manage its effects. Cooking vegetables thoroughly and peeling fruits can make fiber easier to digest.

## Hydration and its Role in Gut Health

Hydration is essential for anyone with EPI, as it helps the digestive system function more smoothly and prevents issues like constipation, which can be common due to malabsorption. Aim to drink plenty of water throughout the day, especially before and after meals, to help with the breakdown and absorption of nutrients.

In addition to water, herbal teas like ginger or peppermint can aid digestion, soothing the gut and reducing bloating or discomfort. Be cautious with sugary drinks, caffeinated beverages, or carbonated drinks, which can irritate the stomach and lead to gas and bloating. Electrolyte-rich beverages may also help maintain balance if you're experiencing dehydration due to malabsorption.

## Vitamins and Minerals for Pancreatic Support

People with EPI often experience deficiencies in fat-soluble vitamins (A, D, E, K) due to difficulty absorbing fats. Incorporating these vitamins into your diet is important, but you should also ensure you're taking them with enzyme supplements to aid absorption. Vitamin D, in particular, is crucial for maintaining bone health, especially in individuals with EPI, as they may suffer from malnutrition.

Minerals such as magnesium and zinc support immune function and overall health. Include foods like leafy greens, nuts, seeds, and fortified cereals in your meals, and consider taking supplements if recommended by your healthcare provider. Always pair vitamin and mineral intake with proper enzyme supplementation to maximize absorption and improve health outcomes.

# Chapter 2:

# Best Grocery Store Foods to Stockpile

## Choosing Low-FODMAP and Easily Digestible Foods

When managing Exocrine Pancreatic Insufficiency (EPI), choosing low-FODMAP and easily digestible foods is essential for reducing gut discomfort. Low-FODMAP foods, such as bananas, carrots, zucchini, and potatoes, help minimize bloating and gas, making them ideal for EPI patients. Focus on simple carbohydrates like rice and gluten-free bread, which are gentle on the digestive system and easy to absorb. Avoid high-FODMAP foods like garlic, onions, and certain beans, which can trigger bloating and discomfort.

To make digestion easier, opt for cooked or steamed vegetables rather than raw, and peel fruits to reduce fiber content. Smoothies made with low-FODMAP fruits like berries, spinach, and lactose-free yogurt are great options. When cooking, use methods like steaming, boiling, or roasting to retain nutrients while making foods easier to digest, promoting overall gut health and comfort.

# Ideal Protein Sources for EPI

Lean proteins are crucial for those with EPI because they are easier to digest and provide essential nutrients. Ideal protein sources include skinless chicken, turkey, and white fish like cod or haddock. These proteins are low in fat, reducing the strain on your pancreas. Eggs (especially egg whites) are another excellent option, as they offer high-quality protein without adding unnecessary fat.

For plant-based proteins, consider tofu, lentils, and chickpeas, which are gentler on the digestive system than other legumes. Cook lentils and chickpeas thoroughly to improve digestibility, and pair them with low-FODMAP grains like quinoa. Incorporating these proteins into your meals supports muscle maintenance and overall health while keeping pancreatic strain to a minimum.

# Healthy Fats and Oils

For EPI management, it's important to incorporate healthy fats and oils that are easier to digest. Opt for medium-chain triglycerides (MCTs), found in coconut oil, which are rapidly absorbed and used by the body, bypassing the need for pancreatic enzymes. Olive oil is another great choice, as it provides heart-healthy monounsaturated fats without overwhelming the digestive system. Use these oils for cooking or as dressings to boost nutrient absorption without causing digestive distress.

Avoid trans fats and high-fat processed foods like fried snacks, which are difficult to digest and can worsen EPI symptoms. Instead, include small portions of avocado or nut butter in your meals for a balanced fat intake. Moderation is key, as even healthy fats should be consumed in controlled amounts to prevent digestive overload.

## Low-Sugar and Low-Sodium Options

Reducing sugar and sodium intake is vital for individuals with EPI to avoid digestive irritation and maintain overall health. Choose natural sweeteners like stevia or monk fruit in place of refined sugars to prevent blood sugar spikes. When selecting packaged foods, look for labels with minimal added sugars, and opt for fruits like berries, which are naturally lower in sugar but still flavorful.

When it comes to sodium, opt for fresh herbs, garlic-infused oil, or lemon juice to season your meals instead of relying on salt-heavy condiments or processed foods. Low-sodium broths and homemade soups using fresh ingredients are excellent alternatives to canned options. This approach supports not only digestive health but also heart health, which is crucial for EPI patients.

## Convenient and Gut-Friendly Snacks

For convenient, gut-friendly snacks, focus on easily digestible, nutrient-rich options that won't trigger symptoms. Rice cakes with a spread of almond butter, lactose-free yogurt with blueberries, or boiled eggs are simple and nutritious choices. These snacks are light yet satisfying, offering protein and energy without overloading your digestive system.

Another great option is homemade smoothies made with lactose-free milk or almond milk, a handful of spinach, and low-FODMAP fruits like strawberries or kiwi. Keep pre-prepared snacks like hard-boiled eggs or portioned nuts on hand for quick, healthy options. These snacks help maintain energy levels throughout the day while supporting gut health.

# Chapter 3:

# Appetizers

## Simple and Nourishing Starters

For individuals with Exocrine Pancreatic Insufficiency (EPI), starters need to be easy on the digestive system while providing essential nutrients. A great example is a soft scrambled egg dish made with lactose-free cheese and a dash of olive oil, which offers a smooth texture that's easy to digest and rich in protein. Another option is mashed avocado spread on gluten-free toast. The healthy fats from avocado support digestion, and when mashed finely, it reduces strain on the digestive system.

Another simple starter could be a small portion of baked sweet potato. High in fiber and gentle on the gut, sweet potatoes provide a nourishing base for EPI management. Serve the sweet potato plain or topped with a small dollop of lactose-free sour cream to make it more enjoyable without upsetting the stomach. The key is to keep ingredients simple and avoid excessive seasoning, which can irritate the pancreas.

## Nutritious Soups and Broths

Nutritious soups and broths are ideal for those with EPI because they are easy to digest and can be packed with nutrients. A bone broth simmered for hours releases collagen and amino acids, promoting gut healing and aiding digestion. It's best served warm and sipped slowly to support gentle digestion. Alternatively, a simple vegetable soup made with carrots, zucchini, and butternut squash is a great option. These vegetables are naturally soft and become even easier to digest after cooking.

To prepare, simply simmer chopped vegetables in low-sodium chicken or vegetable broth until they are soft enough to blend into a smooth soup. This creates a creamy texture without needing heavy cream or butter, which can be hard on the pancreas. A pinch of turmeric or ginger can be added for anti-inflammatory benefits, but keep spices mild to avoid any digestive discomfort.

## Easy-to-Digest Dips and Spreads

Dips and spreads can be nourishing and easy on the stomach when chosen carefully. A great EPI-friendly option is a smooth hummus made from cooked chickpeas, tahini, and olive oil. The key is to blend it to a fine consistency, which makes it easier to digest while providing a good source of plant-based protein and fiber. You can serve it with lightly steamed veggies like carrot sticks or cucumber slices for added nutrition without causing stress on the digestive system.

Another simple dip is a yogurt-based spread made with lactose-free Greek yogurt and a touch of dill or cucumber for flavor. The yogurt provides probiotics that aid in gut health, while the smooth texture makes it ideal for those managing EPI. Be sure to choose lactose-free products and avoid using too much garlic or onion, as these can trigger symptoms.

## Light Vegetable-Based Appetizers

For vegetable-based appetizers, choose ingredients that are naturally low in fiber and easy to digest, such as zucchini, carrots, or bell peppers. Lightly steaming or roasting these vegetables makes them even gentler on the gut. A simple dish like steamed zucchini slices with a drizzle of olive oil and a sprinkle of sea salt is both light and nourishing. It's easy to prepare and won't overwhelm the digestive system.

Another option is roasted carrots or bell peppers served with a small side of lactose-free yogurt dipping sauce. The roasting process softens the vegetables, making them easier to chew and digest while enhancing their natural sweetness. These light appetizers can be filling without causing digestive discomfort, perfect for those with EPI looking to enjoy vegetables in a manageable way.

## Protein-Rich Options for EPI

Protein is essential for maintaining muscle mass and overall health, especially for those with EPI. A simple, protein-rich option is baked or grilled fish, such as salmon or cod, which provides lean protein and healthy fats that are easy to digest. Fish should be cooked, using gentle methods like baking or steaming, and seasoned with herbs like parsley or lemon to avoid irritating the digestive system. Serve with a side of steamed vegetables or a small serving of quinoa.

Another protein-rich option is scrambled eggs with lactose-free cheese. Eggs are soft, easy to digest, and can be cooked quickly with minimal oil. Avoid adding heavy ingredients like butter or cream, as these can trigger symptoms. Instead, prepare the eggs lightly with olive oil and serve with a side of mashed avocado or soft vegetables like sautéed spinach. This ensures a balanced, protein-packed meal that supports digestion and provides essential nutrients.

Chapter 4: Breakfast

## Quick and Easy Breakfast Ideas

When managing Exocrine Pancreatic Insufficiency (EPI), starting the day with simple, gut-friendly breakfasts is key. One quick idea is scrambled eggs with sautéed spinach. The eggs provide easy-to-digest protein, while spinach adds fiber and nutrients without irritating the gut. Another option is a smoothie bowl using lactose-free yogurt, blended with soft fruits like bananas and blueberries, and topped with a sprinkle of chia seeds for extra fiber and omega-3s.

A second quick idea is avocado toast on gluten-free bread. The healthy fats in avocado support digestion, while gluten-free bread helps reduce inflammation for those sensitive to wheat. You can top it with a poached egg for added protein. These breakfasts can be prepared in under 10 minutes, making them convenient and beneficial for digestion.

## Digestive-Friendly Smoothies

Smoothies are perfect for EPI because they're easy on the digestive system. Start with a lactose-free or plant-based milk base, like almond or oat milk, and add fruits such as ripe bananas or berries, which are gentle on the gut. To boost digestion, incorporate a small piece of fresh ginger or a spoonful of flaxseeds. These ingredients support enzyme production and promote gut health.

To keep things balanced, add a handful of spinach for fiber and a spoonful of nut butter for healthy fats. Protein powders like collagen or pea protein can also be blended in to help meet your daily protein needs without stressing the pancreas. Blend everything until smooth, and you have a quick, digestion-friendly meal on the go.

## Protein-Packed Breakfast Options

Protein is essential for those with EPI, but choosing easy-to-digest sources is important. A great option is Greek yogurt with a drizzle of honey and some chopped nuts. Greek yogurt is high in protein and, when chosen lactose-free, won't irritate the gut. The nuts provide healthy fats and crunch without overwhelming the digestive system.

Another protein-packed option is a tofu scramble with vegetables. Crumble tofu into a pan with some olive oil and sauté it with gut-friendly veggies like zucchini and bell peppers. Season with turmeric and a pinch of salt. This breakfast is not only high in protein but also contains antioxidants from the veggies, making it a complete, balanced meal.

## Low-FODMAP and Low-Sugar Recipes

For EPI, low-FODMAP and low-sugar breakfasts help avoid digestive upset. A simple low-FODMAP breakfast option is a chia pudding made with almond milk. Soak chia seeds overnight in almond milk with a pinch of cinnamon for flavor. In the morning, top it with fresh strawberries or blueberries, which are both low in FODMAPs and sugar.

Another option is a veggie omelet made with eggs, spinach, and tomatoes. These ingredients are low-FODMAP and easy to digest, providing essential nutrients without overloading the pancreas. Avoid high-FODMAP ingredients like onions or garlic, which can cause bloating and discomfort. This omelet is a perfect low-sugar, high-protein meal to start the day.

## Nutritious Oatmeal and Porridges

Oatmeal is a great breakfast option for EPI when prepared with care. Use gluten-free oats and cook them in almond or lactose-free milk for a creamy texture. Stir in a tablespoon of chia seeds for extra fiber and omega-3s, and top with sliced bananas for a natural sweetness that's easy on digestion. This combination supports digestive health while providing sustained energy.

If you prefer savory porridge, try a rice porridge (congee) made with bone broth. Cook the rice slowly until it breaks down into a smooth texture.

# Chapter 5:

# Lunch

## Balanced and Easy-to-Digest Lunches

To create easy-to-digest lunches for those managing Exocrine Pancreatic Insufficiency (EPI), focus on meals that are gentle on the stomach but still packed with essential nutrients. A simple grilled chicken and steamed vegetable bowl, for example, provides lean protein and fiber without causing digestive discomfort. Pair this with a small serving of brown rice or quinoa to add energy-sustaining carbohydrates, and avoid excessive oils or spices that may irritate the digestive tract.

Another option is a turkey and avocado wrap made with a gluten-free tortilla. Turkey is a lean protein, and avocado offers healthy fats that support digestion. Add cucumber and spinach for extra vitamins and crunch. Make sure to include a digestive enzyme supplement with these meals to ensure proper nutrient absorption, a key consideration for those with EPI.

## Nutrient-Rich Salads

For nutrient-rich salads that are easy on the digestive system, use a base of leafy greens like spinach or romaine, which are less fibrous and easier to digest than tougher greens like kale. Top with simple, digestible ingredients such as shredded carrots, boiled eggs, or grilled salmon.

These foods provide vitamins, healthy fats, and protein, which are essential for maintaining energy and health while managing EPI.

Dress the salad lightly with olive oil and lemon juice, avoiding heavy or creamy dressings that can cause digestive strain. To add a bit of texture and flavor, sprinkle in some sunflower seeds or flaxseeds, which offer healthy fats and fiber without being too harsh on the gut. Remember to consume enzyme supplements with your meal to aid in nutrient breakdown.

## Hearty and Gentle Soups

Soups are an excellent choice for managing EPI because they are easy to digest and can be loaded with nutrients. A chicken and vegetable soup made with bone broth can provide essential minerals and amino acids that are gentle on the stomach. Use soft vegetables like zucchini, carrots, and spinach, which break down easily during cooking and won't irritate the gut. Avoid beans or cruciferous vegetables like broccoli, as these can be more difficult to digest.

For added protein, include shredded chicken or turkey, and be mindful to avoid cream-based soups, which might be too rich for those with EPI. Stick with clear broths or light coconut milk for a gentler alternative. Pureeing the soup can also make it even easier to digest and absorb, which is essential when managing pancreatic insufficiency.

## Simple Grain and Protein Bowls

Grain and protein bowls can be customized to suit both your nutritional needs and your digestive comfort. Start with a base of easy-to-digest grains like white rice, quinoa, or millet. These grains are gentle on the stomach while providing essential carbohydrates for energy. Pair the grains with lean proteins like grilled chicken, tofu, or soft-cooked fish, which offer easily absorbable amino acids without burdening the digestive system.

Top the bowl with soft, cooked vegetables like sweet potatoes, spinach, or carrots. These vegetables are packed with vitamins and minerals but are soft enough to digest without causing bloating or discomfort. Adding a drizzle of olive oil or a sprinkle of herbs can enhance flavor without overwhelming the gut, making it an ideal, nutrient-dense meal for someone managing EPI.

## Low-FODMAP Sandwiches and Wraps

Low-FODMAP sandwiches and wraps can help ease digestive symptoms for those with EPI by reducing the intake of hard-to-digest sugars and fibers. Opt for gluten-free bread or low-FODMAP wraps, and fill them with lean proteins like turkey, chicken, or firm tofu. These proteins are low in FODMAPs and easy to digest. Add cucumber, lettuce, or thinly sliced bell peppers for crunch and nutrition without adding digestive strain.

Skip traditional condiments that may trigger symptoms, like onion or garlic-based spreads, and instead use lactose-free cheese or a small amount of mustard. For extra moisture, avocado can be a great alternative to mayonnaise. Keep your portions moderate and remember to take any prescribed digestive enzymes before eating to ensure proper nutrient absorption.

# Chapter 6:

# Dinner

## Satisfying and Gut-Friendly Dinner Recipes

For individuals managing Exocrine Pancreatic Insufficiency (EPI), gut-friendly dinners should be both comforting and easy on digestion. Focus on lean proteins like chicken or turkey paired with well-cooked, non-cruciferous vegetables like zucchini and carrots. Incorporating healthy fats like olive oil in moderation can enhance nutrient absorption without overwhelming your digestive system. Opt for small, frequent meals to ease the pancreas' workload.

An example of a gut-friendly dinner could be a simple baked chicken breast seasoned with herbs, served with steamed green beans and mashed sweet potatoes. Cooking ingredients until they are soft helps prevent irritation. Pair these dishes with enzyme supplements, if needed, to support digestion, and avoid high-fiber or greasy foods, which can trigger symptoms.

## Easy-to-Digest Protein Dishes

Proteins are essential for maintaining muscle mass and overall health, but with EPI, digestion can be challenging. Select lean sources of protein like fish, chicken, and eggs that are easier to break down. Cooking methods like baking, grilling, or poaching are recommended to reduce added fats and oils, which could slow digestion. Avoid processed meats and fried foods.

A gentle protein option is poached salmon with a squeeze of lemon juice, accompanied by soft, mashed carrots. Salmon is rich in omega-3 fatty acids, which are anti-inflammatory and beneficial for overall health. Be sure to eat small portions to avoid overwhelming the pancreas, and consider using digestive enzyme supplements to aid in protein digestion.

## Light and Nourishing Stews

Stews are an excellent option for those with EPI as they combine easily digestible ingredients in a warming, satisfying dish. A great base for a stew could include low-fat chicken broth, tender vegetables like carrots, zucchini, and peeled potatoes, along with lean proteins such as turkey or chicken. Cooking the ingredients slowly over low heat ensures everything is soft and easy to digest.

A light and nourishing stew recipe could feature diced chicken breast, carrots, and peeled sweet potatoes simmered in broth for a soothing meal. Adding herbs like thyme or parsley can enhance flavor without triggering digestive discomfort. Serve in small portions to minimize digestive strain and support nutrient absorption.

## Vegetable-Based Dinner Options

For EPI-friendly vegetable-based dinners, select non-cruciferous, low-fiber vegetables that are cooked until soft. Zucchini, squash, carrots, and peeled potatoes are good options, as they are less likely to cause gas or bloating. Steam, roast, or sauté these vegetables in small amounts of olive oil for a nutrient-rich yet gentle dish.

A practical example could be roasted zucchini and carrots with a drizzle of olive oil, sprinkled with a little salt and herbs for flavor. Pair these with a small serving of quinoa or white rice to add easily digestible carbohydrates. Cooking the vegetables until tender ensures they won't irritate the digestive system, making for a soothing, plant-based dinner.

## Low-FODMAP and Low-Sugar Entrées

Low-FODMAP and low-sugar entrées are particularly beneficial for those with EPI, as they minimize digestive distress. Opt for proteins like chicken, turkey, or fish, combined with low-FODMAP vegetables such as bell peppers, zucchini, and carrots. Avoid high-sugar sauces or seasonings, and stick to herbs and lemon juice for flavor.

An example of a low-FODMAP, low-sugar entrée is baked cod with roasted zucchini and bell peppers. Cod is a lean, easily digestible fish, while zucchini and peppers provide flavor and nutrients without triggering symptoms. Serve with a side of white rice or quinoa for a balanced meal that's gentle on the gut.

# Chapter 7:

# Desserts

## Healthier Dessert Choices for EPI

When managing Exocrine Pancreatic Insufficiency (EPI), desserts need to be both easy to digest and packed with nutrients. Start by choosing ingredients that support pancreatic health, such as fruits, low-sugar alternatives, and gut-friendly fats. You can swap out processed sugars for natural sweeteners like honey or stevia, which are easier on the digestive system. For example, baked apples with a drizzle of honey provide a sweet, satisfying treat without triggering digestive issues.

Incorporate ingredients rich in fiber and healthy fats, like oats and chia seeds, to make desserts that aid digestion and provide energy. A simple chia pudding made with coconut milk and sweetened with a bit of maple syrup is a perfect example of a nutritious dessert for someone with EPI. These desserts not only taste great but also help manage symptoms and boost digestive health.

## Simple Fruit-Based Desserts

Fruit-based desserts are ideal for people with EPI because they are naturally sweet, light, and packed with vitamins. Try making a quick fruit salad using easy-to-digest options like bananas, blueberries, and melons, which won't overwhelm the digestive system. Add a squeeze of lemon juice and a sprinkle of mint for an extra burst of flavor without the need for added sugar.

Another simple option is baking fruits like pears or peaches, which enhances their natural sweetness and makes them easier to digest. You can bake them with a sprinkle of cinnamon and a dollop of coconut yogurt on top for added creaminess without the dairy, creating a delicious and gut-friendly dessert.

## Light and Nutritious Puddings

For a light yet filling dessert, puddings made with simple ingredients can offer a great balance of taste and nutrition. A chia seed pudding, for instance, is easy to make by mixing chia seeds with almond or coconut milk, allowing them to soak and thicken overnight. Add a bit of vanilla extract or cinnamon to enhance the flavor, and you've got a creamy dessert that's gentle on the digestive system.

You can also create a rice pudding using low-fat milk or a dairy-free option like oat milk. By keeping the sugar content low and incorporating spices like nutmeg or cardamom, this pudding becomes a soothing and nutritious dessert that won't aggravate EPI symptoms.

## Low-Sugar and Low-FODMAP Treats

For those managing EPI and also sensitive to FODMAPs, low-sugar, low-FODMAP treats can still satisfy a sweet tooth without causing discomfort. Opt for sweeteners like stevia or monk fruit, which don't spike blood sugar or irritate digestion. A good example is a low-sugar coconut macaron, made with unsweetened shredded coconut, egg whites, and stevia, baked until golden.

FODMAP-friendly fruits like strawberries or kiwi can also be used in desserts such as strawberry sorbet. Simply blend the fruit with a bit of lemon juice and freeze until solid. This light and refreshing dessert offers a burst of flavor without triggering digestive issues common with higher FODMAP ingredients.

## Dairy-Free Dessert Options

Dairy can be a major issue for people with EPI, so opting for dairy-free dessert options is essential. Coconut-based products are a fantastic alternative, offering a creamy texture without the lactose. Try making dairy-free ice cream by blending frozen bananas with coconut milk and a dash of vanilla extract for a creamy, indulgent dessert that's easy on the stomach.

Another option is making a dairy-free chocolate mousse using avocado as the base. Simply blend ripe avocados with cocoa powder and a touch of maple syrup until smooth. This rich, velvety dessert is packed with healthy fats that are easier to digest and support overall gut health.

# Chapter 8:

# Vegetarian Recipes

## Digestive-Friendly Vegetarian Meals

Creating vegetarian meals that are easy on the digestive system is essential for those managing Exocrine Pancreatic Insufficiency (EPI). Focus on cooking with easily digestible vegetables like carrots, zucchini, and spinach, which are gentle on the gut. Steaming or lightly roasting these vegetables helps to retain their nutrients while making them softer for digestion. Pair them with healthy fats like olive oil or avocado to aid in nutrient absorption. Avoid using raw vegetables, which can be hard on the digestive system, and instead opt for cooked versions to support easier digestion.

Incorporating foods like sweet potatoes, squash, and pumpkin can provide a soothing base for meals. These starchy vegetables are rich in fiber but gentle on the stomach, helping to promote healthy digestion. Consider creating soups or purees that blend these ingredients for a nourishing and simple meal. Use herbs like ginger and turmeric, which are known to promote gut health, making them perfect for flavoring your dishes while offering additional digestive benefits.

# Protein-Rich Plant-Based Dishes

For those with EPI, it's important to include plant-based proteins that are easy to digest. Options such as tofu, tempeh, and lentils provide a rich source of protein without overloading the digestive system. Tofu and tempeh can be cooked in various ways—baked, grilled, or sautéed with light seasoning. For example, marinate tofu in a small amount of soy sauce and bake it until golden for a protein-packed meal that supports digestive health.

Lentils, particularly red and yellow varieties, are softer and easier to digest compared to beans. Boil them with mild spices like cumin and coriander to create a flavorful stew or curry that's light on the stomach. Pairing plant proteins with gentle grains like quinoa or rice helps create a balanced, protein-rich meal that supports overall digestion while providing essential nutrients.

## Low-FODMAP Vegetarian Options

For those managing EPI, following a low-FODMAP diet can significantly reduce bloating and discomfort. Opt for low-FODMAP vegetables like bell peppers, zucchini, and spinach, which are gentle on the digestive system. You can roast or sauté these vegetables in olive oil for a simple, gut-friendly side dish. Low-FODMAP grains such as rice or quinoa serve as great bases for meals and can be paired with vegetables for a complete, easy-to-digest dish.

To make a low-FODMAP meal more satisfying, add lactose-free cheeses or a drizzle of olive oil for flavor. Consider making a stir-fry with zucchini, bell peppers, and firm tofu, seasoned with a low-FODMAP sauce like soy sauce or ginger. This combination provides essential nutrients while being easy to digest, making it a great option for those dealing with digestive issues.

## Nutritious and Simple Vegetable Recipes

Nutritious vegetable recipes for EPI management should focus on simple preparation methods that preserve vitamins while being gentle on the gut. Steamed carrots, spinach, and green beans are excellent choices as they are easy to digest and packed with essential nutrients like fiber, and vitamins A and C. Drizzling a little olive oil over these veggies before serving can enhance flavor and nutrient absorption without causing digestive discomfort.

You can also make simple, one-pot vegetable soups using ingredients like carrots, zucchini, and butternut squash. Simmer these vegetables in a light vegetable broth and blend into a smooth puree. This creates a soothing, nourishing meal that is rich in fiber and vitamins while being very gentle on the digestive system, ideal for those dealing with EPI symptoms.

## Easy-to-Digest Meat Alternatives

Easy-to-digest meat alternatives like tofu, tempeh, and eggs are excellent options for managing EPI. Tofu and tempeh can be marinated in light seasonings and grilled or baked to create a satisfying and nutritious protein source. Scrambled eggs are another simple option that can be quickly prepared and are easy on the digestive system, making them perfect for a light meal.

If you're looking for something heartier, try making a tofu stir-fry with low-FODMAP vegetables such as zucchini and spinach. Sauté the tofu with a little olive oil and add in the vegetables for a complete meal that is both nourishing and easy to digest. For those looking for more variety, try quinoa as a protein-packed base for dishes, or soft-cooked eggs with lightly sautéed greens for a simple, EPI-friendly breakfast.

# Chapter 9:

# Snacking Strategies

## Healthy and Gut-Friendly Snack Ideas

For those managing EPI, snacks need to be gentle on the digestive system while providing essential nutrients. Focus on easily digestible snacks like banana slices with almond butter, yogurt with low-fiber fruits (like blueberries), or smoothies made with lactose-free milk and protein powders. These snacks are easy on the pancreas, support digestion, and help reduce inflammation. Incorporating protein and healthy fats is essential to maintain energy levels and support gut health.

You can also prepare simple gut-friendly snacks like boiled eggs, soft cheese, or avocado spread on gluten-free crackers. Pairing high-protein items with small amounts of healthy fats aids in nutrient absorption while keeping digestion manageable. Remember to avoid heavy, fried, or processed foods, as they can cause digestive discomfort.

## Easy-to-Make and Portable Snacks

When you're on the go, quick and portable snacks are a lifesaver. Prepare small, easy-to-carry options like hard-boiled eggs, individual servings of lactose-free yogurt, or pre-portioned nuts. You can also create small snack packs with sliced cucumber, carrot sticks, and a protein dip like hummus or lactose-free cottage cheese.

If you need something more filling, try making portable protein smoothies using gut-friendly ingredients such as lactose-free milk, plant-based protein powder, and low-sugar fruits like berries. Store them in small containers so they're ready when you need them. These snacks are easy to pack and digest, making them perfect for anyone managing EPI.

## Nutrient-Dense Snack Options

When dealing with EPI, it's essential to pack your snacks with as many nutrients as possible. Nut butter spread on rice cakes or paired with a small apple provides healthy fats and carbohydrates. You could also try energy balls made from oats, nut butter, and a low-sugar sweetener like honey for a balanced, nutrient-dense treat.

For a more substantial option, you can prepare mini turkey or chicken wraps using gluten-free tortillas and add some avocado or spinach for extra vitamins. These nutrient-dense snacks provide essential protein, fats, and fiber, all while being gentle on your digestive system and easy to prepare.

## Low-FODMAP and Low-Sugar Choices

For EPI-friendly snacks that are also low-FODMAP, opt for items like rice crackers with lactose-free cheese, or carrot sticks with a dollop of peanut butter. These snacks help avoid gut irritants like excess fiber or fermentable carbs, which can worsen symptoms. Low-FODMAP choices are ideal for supporting digestion while avoiding bloating and discomfort.

Low-sugar snacks, such as a handful of unsweetened nuts or chia pudding made with coconut milk, are perfect for maintaining stable blood sugar levels. They offer a steady energy release without triggering insulin spikes, which can be a concern for those managing pancreatic health issues.

## Balancing Snacks for Digestive Health

Balancing your snacks with the right mix of protein, fats, and carbs can help optimize digestion for those with EPI. Combining lactose-free Greek yogurt with a handful of berries offers probiotics for gut health, along with balanced nutrients. Another example is pairing apple slices with almond butter, offering both fiber and healthy fats to help the body absorb vitamins more effectively.

When choosing snacks, always consider pairing a lean protein with a healthy fat to enhance nutrient absorption. For instance, mix a small portion of lean turkey slices with avocado or pair gluten-free crackers with a hard-boiled egg to provide energy while being easy on your digestive system.

# Chapter 10:

# Smoothies

## Digestive-Friendly Smoothie Recipes

For those managing Exocrine Pancreatic Insufficiency (EPI), digestive-friendly smoothies can provide relief and nourishment. Start with a base of low-fiber ingredients like ripe bananas or cooked apples, which are gentle on the digestive system. Blend these with plain yogurt or almond milk to create a smooth, easily digestible mixture. Avoid high-fiber or gas-inducing ingredients like raw vegetables and fruits with tough skins. For added flavor and nutrition, incorporate mild spices like cinnamon or a small amount of vanilla extract.

Additionally, consider adding digestive aids such as ginger or turmeric. These ingredients not only enhance flavor but also support digestive health. For a balanced smoothie, include a small amount of honey or a low-FODMAP sweetener. Aim for a texture that's smooth and creamy to ensure it's easy on your digestive system. Always test new ingredients in small amounts to gauge your tolerance.

## Nutrient-Packed Blends for EPI

Nutrient-packed blends are essential for those with EPI to ensure they receive adequate vitamins and minerals despite dietary restrictions. Use nutrient-dense fruits like blueberries and strawberries, which are rich in antioxidants but gentle on the stomach. Combine these with spinach or kale, which provide essential vitamins without being overly fibrous if used in small amounts. Opt for a base like kefir or a lactose-free milk alternative to enhance nutrient absorption and gut health.

Incorporate protein sources like whey protein powder or a plant-based protein blend to support overall health and muscle maintenance. Consider adding a spoonful of chia seeds or flaxseeds for omega-3 fatty acids, which can support inflammation control and digestion. Blend ingredients thoroughly to avoid any gritty texture and ensure smoothness.

## Low-FODMAP and Low-Sugar Smoothies

Low-FODMAP and low-sugar smoothies are ideal for managing EPI while minimizing digestive discomfort. Start with low-FODMAP fruits such as strawberries, blueberries, and kiwi, and avoid high-FODMAP fruits like apples and pears. Use unsweetened almond milk or coconut water as a base to keep sugar content low and prevent digestive upset.

Incorporate a small amount of low-FODMAP vegetables like cucumbers or carrots, which are less likely to cause bloating. For sweetness, use a small amount of a low-FODMAP sweetener like maple syrup or stevia. Blending these ingredients until smooth will help ensure that the smoothie remains gentle on the digestive system while still providing necessary nutrients.

## Protein-Boosted Smoothie Options

Protein-boosted smoothies are an excellent choice for individuals with EPI to ensure they are getting enough protein in their diet. Start with a base of protein-rich options like Greek yogurt, cottage cheese, or a protein powder that suits your dietary needs. Combine these with easily digestible fruits such as bananas or berries for added flavor and nutrients.

To further increase protein content, consider adding a tablespoon of nut butter or hemp seeds. These ingredients are not only protein-rich but also provide healthy fats that can be beneficial for energy and overall health. Blend all ingredients until the mixture is smooth to ensure easy digestion and avoid any chunky or gritty texture.

## Hydrating and Nourishing Smoothie Ideas

Hydrating and nourishing smoothies can support overall health and digestion for those managing EPI. Use hydrating ingredients such as cucumber, coconut water, or melon, which help maintain fluid balance and provide gentle nourishment. Combining these with greens like spinach or kale in small quantities can enhance nutrient content without adding excess fiber.

For added nourishment, include ingredients rich in essential fatty acids, such as chia seeds or avocado, which can help with inflammation and overall health. Blend these ingredients until smooth to ensure the smoothie is easy on the digestive system and provides both hydration and nourishment. Always adjust ingredient quantities based on individual tolerance levels.

# Chapter 11:

# Soup Recipes

## Healing and Gentle Soups

Healing and gentle soups are essential for individuals with Exocrine Pancreatic Insufficiency (EPI), as they provide nourishment without straining the digestive system. To make a healing soup, start by using low-fat bone broth or vegetable broth as a base, which is easy on the stomach and helps soothe digestive discomfort. Incorporate ingredients like well-cooked carrots, celery, and squash, which are easily digestible and rich in nutrients. Blend the soup until smooth to eliminate any potential fiber that might be hard to digest.

For added benefits, consider including a small amount of ginger or turmeric, both known for their anti-inflammatory properties. Ensure that all ingredients are thoroughly cooked and well-blended to maintain a gentle texture that supports digestive health. Avoid using raw vegetables or high-fat ingredients, as these can exacerbate symptoms.

## Protein-Rich Soup Options

Protein-rich soups are vital for managing EPI because they support muscle maintenance and overall health. Opt for lean proteins like chicken breast or turkey, which should be cooked thoroughly and shredded or finely chopped before adding to your soup. For a simple recipe, simmer diced chicken breast in low-sodium chicken broth with a few soft vegetables such as zucchini or green beans. Blend the mixture to a smooth consistency to make it easier on your digestive system.

Another excellent protein source is well-cooked legumes like lentils or split peas, though these should be used cautiously due to their fiber content. If tolerated, blend them into a creamy soup with a base of vegetable broth. Always ensure that the soup is strained or blended to minimize any undigested particles.

## Vegetable-Based Soups for EPI

Vegetable-based soups can be very beneficial for EPI when prepared properly. Start with a base of low-sodium vegetable broth and add vegetables like carrots, spinach, and pumpkin, which are gentle on the digestive system. Cook the vegetables until they are very soft and then blend the soup to achieve a smooth texture, making it easier for your body to process.

Avoid using cruciferous vegetables like broccoli or cauliflower, as they may cause gas or bloating. Instead, focus on easily digestible vegetables and season lightly with herbs such as basil or thyme for added flavor without overwhelming the digestive system.

## Low-FODMAP Soup Recipes

Low-FODMAP soups are designed to minimize symptoms associated with EPI by avoiding high-fermentable carbohydrates that can cause digestive issues. Use a base of low-sodium chicken or vegetable broth and include ingredients like carrots, spinach, and potatoes. Ensure all ingredients are well-cooked and blended to reduce their fermentable content.

For flavor, use fresh herbs like parsley or cilantro instead of high-FODMAP ingredients such as onions and garlic. Always monitor your body's response to new ingredients to ensure they are well-tolerated and make adjustments as needed.

## Easy and Quick Soup Ideas

For quick and easy soups, focus on simple recipes that require minimal preparation. Use pre-cooked or canned low-sodium broths as a base and add quick-cooking vegetables like spinach or baby carrots. To boost protein, incorporate rotisserie chicken or pre-cooked tofu, ensuring these ingredients are cut into small, digestible pieces.

An easy recipe is a basic chicken and spinach soup: heat low-sodium chicken broth, add shredded rotisserie chicken, and stir in fresh spinach until wilted. Blend if necessary to achieve a smooth consistency. This type of soup can be prepared in under 30 minutes, making it both practical and gentle on your digestive system.

# Chapter 12:

# Salad Recipes

## Nutritious and Digestive-Friendly Salads

Creating salads that are gentle on the digestive system is crucial for managing EPI. Opt for leafy greens like spinach or romaine, which are high in fiber but easy to digest. Incorporate ingredients like shredded carrots, cucumbers, and bell peppers for added nutrients without overwhelming your gut. Avoid high-fat or raw cruciferous vegetables such as broccoli or cabbage, as they may exacerbate symptoms.

For a digestive boost, include ingredients like cooked quinoa or lentils, which provide beneficial fiber and protein without being harsh on the stomach. Ensure that all vegetables are well-washed and cut into small, manageable pieces to enhance digestibility. For added flavor and nutrients, consider incorporating herbs such as parsley or cilantro.

## Protein-Packed Salad Ideas

Protein is vital for individuals with EPI to support digestive health and overall well-being. Include easily digestible protein sources like grilled chicken breast, baked tofu, or canned tuna. These options are not only nutrient-dense but also gentle on the stomach, making them ideal for EPI management.

To further enhance your salad, add a side of cooked beans or legumes like chickpeas, which are rich in protein and fiber. Avoid heavy or fried proteins that can be hard on digestion. Ensure the protein is well-cooked and shredded or chopped into small pieces for easier digestion and absorption.

## Low-FODMAP Salad Recipes

For individuals with EPI, low-FODMAP ingredients can help manage digestive symptoms. Use ingredients such as spinach, cucumbers, and carrots, which are low in fermentable oligosaccharides, disaccharides, monosaccharides, and polyols (FODMAPs). Avoid high-FODMAP ingredients like onions, garlic, and certain legumes.

Incorporate low-FODMAP fruits like strawberries or blueberries for a touch of sweetness. Always check portion sizes to ensure they remain within low-FODMAP limits. By focusing on these ingredients, you can create salads that are both satisfying and easy on the digestive system.

## Simple and Fresh Salad Dressings

Creating salad dressings that are both flavorful and easy on the stomach is essential. Opt for simple dressings made with ingredients like olive oil, lemon juice, and herbs. For example, a basic vinaigrette made with olive oil, apple cider vinegar, and a pinch of salt can enhance the flavor of your salad without causing digestive discomfort.

Avoid dressings that contain cream or high-fat ingredients, as these can exacerbate EPI symptoms. For added flavor, consider using fresh herbs like basil or dill, which are gentle on the digestive system and can add a burst of freshness to your salads.

## Balanced Salad Bowls for EPI

Balanced salad bowls combine a variety of nutrient-dense ingredients that support digestive health. Start with a base of leafy greens, then add a source of protein like grilled chicken or tofu, and include cooked grains such as quinoa. Incorporate a variety of vegetables like cucumbers, bell peppers, and carrots for added nutrients.

For a balanced approach, include a small portion of healthy fats such as avocado or seeds. Avoid ingredients that are high in fat or raw vegetables that may be difficult to digest. Combine these components into a well-rounded bowl that supports digestion and provides essential nutrients for managing EPI symptoms.

# Chapter 13:

# Main Course Recipes

## Easy-to-Digest Main Dishes

For those with Exocrine Pancreatic Insufficiency (EPI), choosing main dishes that are gentle on the digestive system is crucial. Opt for recipes that use lean meats like chicken or turkey, as these are easier to break down. Cooking methods like baking, steaming, or slow-cooking can help retain the nutrients while making the food softer and easier to digest. For example, a baked chicken breast with a side of steamed carrots provides a simple, gentle meal that's both nourishing and easy on the stomach.

Incorporate easily digestible grains such as white rice or quinoa into your meals. These grains are less likely to cause digestive discomfort compared to whole grains. A mild, low-fat chicken and rice casserole can be a perfect main dish. Just ensure the recipe avoids high-fat ingredients and includes well-cooked vegetables that are soft and easy to digest.

## Protein-Rich and Gentle Entrees

When managing EPI, incorporating protein-rich foods that are easy on the stomach is key. Choose proteins like eggs, tofu, or fish, which are generally well-tolerated and less likely to cause digestive issues. For instance, a poached fish fillet served with a side of well-cooked spinach can offer a high-protein, low-fat meal that's gentle on the digestive tract.

Another good option is a tofu stir-fry with mild vegetables. Tofu provides a high-quality protein source that's easy to digest, and cooking it with soft vegetables in a gentle sauce ensures that the meal remains easy on the stomach while still providing essential nutrients.

## Low-FODMAP Main Course Options

Low-FODMAP diets are beneficial for those with EPI, as they can reduce symptoms by avoiding fermentable oligosaccharides, disaccharides, monosaccharides, and polyols. Opt for recipes that include low-FODMAP vegetables like carrots, zucchini, and bell peppers. A low-FODMAP chicken and vegetable soup, made with these ingredients and a low-sodium broth, is a practical and soothing meal option.

Quinoa and lean meats are also suitable for a low-FODMAP diet. A simple quinoa and grilled chicken bowl with steamed spinach and a sprinkle of fresh herbs provides a balanced, gut-friendly meal that aligns with EPI dietary needs while minimizing discomfort.

## Vegetable-Based Main Dishes

Vegetable-based dishes can be both nutritious and gentle on the stomach if prepared properly. Use well-cooked vegetables that are easy to digest, such as carrots, squash, and spinach. For example, a creamy butternut squash soup, made with low-fat ingredients and blended until smooth, offers a soothing, easily digestible meal option.

Consider making vegetable stews with a focus on low-FODMAP vegetables and avoiding high-fiber or cruciferous vegetables that might cause bloating or discomfort. A simple vegetable stew with potatoes, carrots, and green beans can be both satisfying and gentle on the digestive system.

## Simple and Satisfying Dinner Recipes

For a straightforward and satisfying dinner, aim for meals that are easy to prepare and digest. Recipes that include a balance of lean protein, low-fat carbohydrates, and well-cooked vegetables are ideal. An example is a turkey meatloaf served with mashed sweet potatoes and a side of steamed green beans, providing a comforting and easy-to-digest dinner.

Another practical option is a one-pan-baked dish, such as chicken with roasted carrots and parsnips. This method allows for minimal cleanup while offering a simple, well-balanced meal that's easy on the digestive system and supports pancreatic health.

# Chapter 14:

# Side Dishes

## Digestive-Friendly Side Options

Digestive-friendly side options focus on foods that are gentle on the digestive system, ideal for those managing Exocrine Pancreatic Insufficiency (EPI). To make a soothing side dish, consider steamed vegetables like carrots or zucchini. These vegetables are easy to digest and low in fat, making them suitable for supporting pancreatic health. Prepare them by steaming until tender and seasoning lightly with herbs.

Another option is plain rice or potatoes, which are bland and unlikely to irritate the digestive tract. For instance, boiled white rice provides a soft texture that's easy on the stomach and helps absorb excess stomach acid. Avoid adding heavy sauces or spices that could exacerbate digestive issues.

## Nutrient-Rich Vegetable Sides

Nutrient-rich vegetable sides are essential for providing the vitamins and minerals needed for overall health while managing EPI. Opt for vegetables that are steamed or roasted, such as sweet potatoes, spinach, and green beans. These vegetables are high in essential nutrients and are easy to digest when prepared simply.

For a practical example, you can roast sweet potato cubes with a touch of olive oil and a pinch of salt. This preparation maintains the vegetable's nutritional integrity while being gentle on the digestive system. Including a variety of these nutrient-dense vegetables in your meals ensures you get a balanced intake of vitamins and minerals.

## Simple and Light Grain Side Dishes

Simple and light-grain side dishes help provide energy and are easy on the digestive system. Choose grains like white rice, quinoa, or polenta, which are gentle and less likely to cause digestive discomfort. Cook these grains according to package instructions, using minimal oil and seasoning.

For example, prepare quinoa by rinsing it thoroughly and then cooking it in water or low-sodium broth. This dish is light and easily digestible, making it a great addition to meals for those with EPI. Adding a small amount of cooked spinach or shredded carrots can enhance its nutritional value without overwhelming the digestive system.

## Low-FODMAP and Low-Sugar Sides

Low FODMAP and low-sugar sides are crucial for managing digestive symptoms associated with EPI. Focus on foods that are low in fermentable carbohydrates and sugars to avoid triggering digestive discomfort. Ideal choices include steamed vegetables like bell peppers and cucumbers and fruits such as strawberries.

For instance, make a cucumber salad by slicing cucumbers thinly and tossing them with a little lemon juice and dill. This dish is low in FODMAPs and sugars, making it a suitable side for those with sensitive digestive systems. Always check food labels and recipes to ensure they adhere to low-FODMAP and low-sugar guidelines.

## Protein-Rich Side Dishes

Protein-rich side dishes support muscle health and help maintain energy levels while being gentle on the digestive system. Incorporate lean proteins like grilled chicken breast, eggs, or tofu into your meals. These proteins are less likely to cause digestive issues compared to higher-fat options.

For example, prepare a simple egg dish by scrambling eggs with a bit of spinach or bell pepper. This provides a protein boost and is easy to digest. Another option is grilled chicken breast, seasoned lightly with herbs and served with steamed vegetables. These dishes are nourishing and supportive of overall health while managing EPI.

# Chapter 15:

# Grains and Legumes

## Easy-to-Digest Grain Recipes

For individuals with Exocrine Pancreatic Insufficiency (EPI), easy-to-digest grains are crucial for minimizing digestive discomfort. Opt for grains like white rice, oats, and quinoa, which are less likely to cause bloating and gas. Start with simple recipes such as oatmeal or rice porridge. For oatmeal, cook oats in water or a low-fat milk substitute until soft, and add a pinch of cinnamon for flavor. Ensure the mixture is well-cooked to enhance digestibility.

Another excellent option is white rice. Prepare it by boiling it with a 2:1 water-to-rice ratio until tender. For added nutrients, you can mix in steamed vegetables or a small amount of cooked chicken. Avoid using excessive fats or spices that could exacerbate symptoms. These easy-to-digest grain recipes provide a gentle, supportive base for a gut-friendly diet.

## Low-FODMAP Legume Options

Legumes can be challenging for those with EPI due to their high fiber content and potential to cause gas. However, some legume varieties are better tolerated than others. Opt for low-FODMAP options like lentils and chickpeas, which are easier on the digestive system. For example, cooking lentils thoroughly and serving them in small portions can help reduce digestive strain. A simple recipe involves simmering lentils with turmeric and a pinch of salt until tender, then blending into a smooth soup.

Another practical choice is canned chickpeas, which are pre-cooked and easier to digest. Rinse them thoroughly before use to remove excess sodium and potential irritants. Use them in recipes like a chickpea salad with cucumber and a splash of lemon juice for a refreshing, gut-friendly meal. These options provide essential nutrients while minimizing digestive discomfort.

## Simple and Nutritious Rice Dishes

Rice is a staple that is both versatile and gentle on the stomach. For EPI management, focus on creating simple rice dishes that are easy to digest. One straightforward recipe is rice cooked with chicken broth. Use a 1:2 ratio of rice to broth, and cook until the rice is soft and the broth is absorbed. This dish provides hydration and essential nutrients while being easy on the digestive system.

You can also prepare rice and vegetable pilaf by sautéing finely chopped carrots and peas in a small amount of olive oil before mixing in cooked rice. Season lightly with salt or herbs. This recipe offers a balanced meal with added vitamins and minerals, supporting overall digestive health and comfort.

# Protein-Rich Legume Recipes

For EPI management, incorporating protein-rich legumes can help with maintaining adequate nutrition. A simple and digestible recipe involves making a lentil stew. Cook lentils with carrots, celery, and a small amount of chicken or vegetable broth. Allow the mixture to simmer until the lentils are soft, which helps in easier digestion. For a smoother texture, blend the stew after cooking.

Another option is mung beans, which are known for their digestibility. Prepare them by soaking them overnight and then cooking them until tender. You can mix them into a simple vegetable stir-fry with bell peppers and zucchini. This provides a protein-rich meal that is both nutritious and gentle on the digestive system.

## Balancing Grains and Legumes for EPI

Balancing grains and legumes in your diet is essential for managing EPI while ensuring adequate nutrient intake. Start by combining easily digestible grains, like white rice, with low-FODMAP legumes, such as well-cooked lentils. For example, prepare a dish by mixing cooked rice with a lentil curry, using mild spices and a small amount of olive oil. This combination offers a balanced source of carbohydrates and protein while being gentle on the stomach.

You can also create a grain-legume salad by mixing quinoa with diced, cooked chickpeas and a variety of low-FODMAP vegetables. Dress with a light lemon vinaigrette to enhance flavor without adding irritants. This meal not only provides a balanced nutrient profile but also helps manage EPI symptoms by avoiding high-FODMAP ingredients and focusing on easily digestible options.

# Chapter 16:

# Sauces and Dressings

## Gut-Friendly Sauces and Dressings

T

To create gut-friendly sauces and dressings, focus on ingredients that are gentle on the digestive system and promote pancreatic health. Use bone broths, which are rich in nutrients and easy to digest, as a base for sauces. Incorporate low-FODMAP vegetables like carrots and zucchini, which are less likely to trigger digestive discomfort. Avoid high-fat and spicy ingredients that can exacerbate symptoms of Exocrine Pancreatic Insufficiency (EPI).

For dressings, opt for simple combinations of olive oil, lemon juice, and herbs like basil or parsley. These ingredients are not only soothing but also support pancreatic function. Blend olive oil with a bit of apple cider vinegar and mild herbs for a versatile, digestive-friendly vinaigrette that can be used on salads or as a marinade.

## Low-FODMAP and Low-Sugar Options

Low-FODMAP and low-sugar recipes are ideal for managing EPI symptoms. FODMAPs are a group of fermentable carbohydrates that can cause digestive distress in sensitive individuals. Focus on using low-FODMAP vegetables such as bell peppers, cucumbers, and spinach in your recipes. Replace high-sugar ingredients with natural alternatives like stevia or small amounts of pure maple syrup to avoid aggravating symptoms.

Incorporate low-sugar fruits such as berries and green apples in sauces and dressings for added flavor without high sugar content. For example, a blueberry sauce made with fresh blueberries, a touch of lemon juice, and a low-FODMAP sweetener can provide a delightful addition to dishes while remaining gentle on the gut.

## Easy-to-Make Dressings

Creating easy-to-make dressings is all about using simple ingredients that are readily available and easy on the stomach. For a basic vinaigrette, mix 3 parts olive oil with 1 part apple cider vinegar or lemon juice, and add a pinch of salt. This mixture can be adjusted to taste with mild herbs such as dill or parsley, making it both versatile and soothing for EPI sufferers.

Another simple dressing is a yogurt-based dip, using lactose-free yogurt or a plant-based alternative. Combine yogurt with fresh herbs like chives or cilantro, and a squeeze of lemon juice. This easy dressing can be used for salads or as a vegetable dip, providing a creamy texture without irritating the digestive system.

## Protein-Boosted Sauce Recipes

To boost protein content in sauces, use protein-rich ingredients like collagen powder or egg whites. For example, adding a scoop of unflavored collagen powder to a tomato-based sauce can enhance its protein profile while keeping it mild and gut-friendly. Similarly, a sauce made with blended egg whites and low-FODMAP vegetables can provide a creamy, protein-rich option.

Another method is to incorporate lean meats like chicken breast or turkey into your sauces. Slow-cook shredded chicken with low-FODMAP vegetables and a splash of bone broth for a protein-packed sauce that complements many dishes and supports pancreatic health.

## Simple and Nourishing Sauce Ideas

Simple and nourishing sauces can be made with minimal ingredients while still providing essential nutrients. Try a basic herb sauce by blending fresh herbs such as basil, cilantro, and a small amount of garlic-infused olive oil. This sauce can add flavor without overwhelming the digestive system.

For a creamy, nourishing option, blend cooked butternut squash with a bit of low-sodium vegetable broth and a touch of nutmeg. This squash-based sauce is easy on the stomach, rich in vitamins, and can be used to enhance the flavor of various dishes while supporting digestive health.

# Chapter 17:

# Baking and Bread

## EPI-Friendly Baking Basics

When baking for Exocrine Pancreatic Insufficiency (EPI), focus on low-fat, easily digestible ingredients to minimize pancreatic strain. Opt for whole grains like oats and quinoa, which are gentle on the digestive system and high in fiber. Use unsweetened applesauce or mashed bananas as fat substitutes to keep baked goods moist without adding extra fat. Avoid ingredients high in fat and sugar to maintain digestive comfort and overall health.

## Practical Recipe Example

Try baking a batch of oatmeal cookies using mashed bananas instead of butter. Mix rolled oats with mashed bananas, a touch of cinnamon, and a few chopped nuts or seeds. Form the mixture into cookies and bake until golden. This simple swap reduces fat while maintaining a tasty treat that's easy on your digestive system.

## Understanding Low-FODMAP Ingredients

Low-FODMAP breads are made using ingredients that are less likely to trigger digestive symptoms. Use flour like rice, spelled, or gluten-free blends, which are easier to digest than wheat. Incorporate seeds like chia or flax, which provide fiber without high-FODMAP sugars. Avoid ingredients like honey or high-fructose corn syrup that can exacerbate EPI symptoms.

## Practical Recipe Example

Make a simple gluten-free bread by combining rice flour, almond flour, baking soda, and a pinch of salt. Add a small amount of olive oil and a splash of water to form a dough. Pour into a loaf pan and bake until firm. This bread is not only gentle on the stomach but also provides a satisfying texture without digestive distress.

# Simple and Healthy Muffin Recipes

## Creating Digestive-Friendly Muffins

For muffins that support pancreatic health, use low-fat, low-sugar ingredients. Opt for whole grains or gluten-free flour and incorporate fruits or vegetables for natural sweetness and nutrients. Avoid high-fat ingredients like cream or butter, and use unsweetened yogurt or applesauce instead.

## Practical Recipe Example

Combine whole wheat flour, baking powder, and a pinch of salt in a bowl. Mix in mashed sweet potatoes and a small amount of maple syrup for sweetness. Stir in some blueberries for added flavor and antioxidants. Pour the mixture into muffin tins and bake until a toothpick comes out clean. These muffins are packed with nutrients and are easier on the digestive system.

## Incorporating Protein into Baked Goods

For EPI-friendly protein-packed options, consider adding ingredients like protein powder, nut flour, or seeds to your recipes. Almond flour, chia seeds, and hemp seeds are excellent choices as they provide a protein boost without being overly fatty. Aim to keep overall fat content low to prevent digestive issues.

## Practical Recipe Example

Make protein bars by combining almond flour, protein powder, and a small amount of honey. Mix with chia seeds and a pinch of vanilla extract. Press the mixture into a pan and refrigerate until firm. Cut into bars for a protein-packed snack that supports digestive health without excessive fat.

## Exploring Light Bread Options

For a lighter alternative to traditional bread, use ingredients like almond flour or coconut flour, which are easier to digest and lower in fat. Incorporate vegetables like zucchini or carrots for added moisture and nutrients. Avoid heavy, dense flours that can be hard on the digestive system.

## Practical Recipe Example

Create a light zucchini bread by mixing almond flour, baking powder, and a pinch of salt. Stir in grated zucchini, a touch of olive oil, and a small amount of honey. Pour the batter into a loaf pan and bake until set. This bread alternative provides a soft texture and digestive-friendly nutrients, making it a suitable choice for those managing EPI.

# Chapter 18:

# Cooking Techniques

## Gentle Cooking Methods for EPI

For individuals with Exocrine Pancreatic Insufficiency (EPI), gentle cooking methods are crucial to reduce stress on the digestive system. Steaming, poaching, and slow cooking are ideal as they help retain the nutrients in food while making it easier to digest. For instance, steaming vegetables preserves their vitamins and minerals, making them more beneficial for digestion. Poaching meats in a light broth can help break down proteins, making them easier on the pancreas.

Avoid high-heat cooking methods such as frying or grilling, as these can produce inflammatory compounds that irritate the digestive tract. Instead, use low and slow techniques to prepare meals, which help maintain the food's digestibility and nutritional value. For example, slow-cooked stews or casseroles allow flavors to meld without the need for excessive fats or spices, making them suitable for those managing EPI.

## Best Practices for Cooking Digestive-Friendly Meals

When cooking for EPI, simplicity and mild flavors are key. Focus on using easily digestible ingredients like lean proteins (chicken, turkey) and low-fiber vegetables (carrots, zucchini). Avoid adding heavy sauces or spices that could irritate the digestive system. For example, prepare a simple chicken and vegetable soup by simmering chicken breasts with carrots and celery in a mild broth.

Incorporate small, frequent meals throughout the day rather than large meals to avoid overwhelming the digestive system. Cooking in batches and freezing portions can help manage daily meal planning and ensure you always have gentle, digestive-friendly options on hand. For instance, a batch of plain, poached chicken can be easily added to different meals throughout the week.

## Tips for Reducing FODMAPs in Recipes

Reducing FODMAPs (Fermentable Oligo-, Di-, Mono-saccharides, and Polyols) in recipes helps alleviate digestive discomfort for those with EPI. Focus on using low-FODMAP ingredients such as spinach, bell peppers, and quinoa. For example, replace high-FODMAP garlic and onions with chives or the green parts of scallions in your recipes.

Keep in mind that portion size can impact FODMAP levels, so use moderate amounts of low-FODMAP foods to ensure they don't trigger symptoms. For example, a salad with grilled chicken, bell peppers, and a small amount of feta cheese can be a nutritious and low-FODMAP option. Monitoring your body's response to different foods can help you find what works best for your digestive health.

## Techniques for Enhancing Nutrient Absorption

To enhance nutrient absorption, use methods that maximize the availability of vitamins and minerals in food. Cooking vegetables lightly rather than overcooking them helps preserve their nutrient content. For example, lightly steaming spinach instead of boiling it can retain more of its iron and calcium.

Combining certain foods can also improve nutrient absorption. For instance, pairing iron-rich foods like lean meats with vitamin C-rich vegetables such as bell peppers can enhance iron absorption. Additionally, consuming meals with healthy fats, such as avocado or olive oil, can help absorb fat-soluble vitamins A, D, E, and K more effectively.

## Preparing Meals for Optimal Pancreatic Health

For optimal pancreatic health, focus on low-fat, nutrient-dense meals that are easy to digest. Use lean proteins and whole grains while avoiding high-fat and processed foods. For example, a quinoa and vegetable stir-fry with a small amount of olive oil is a balanced meal that supports pancreatic function.Maintain a balanced ratio of protein, carbohydrates, and fats in your meals to support overall digestion and absorption. Preparing meals with a mix of lean protein (like turkey), complex carbs (like sweet potatoes), and healthy fats (like flaxseed oil) ensures your diet supports pancreatic health without overstressing it. Regularly incorporating these types of meals can help manage EPI symptoms effectively.

# Chapter 19:

# Common Concerns and Detailed FAQs

## Managing Symptoms Through Diet

To effectively manage symptoms of Exocrine Pancreatic Insufficiency (EPI), focus on a diet that is low in fat but high in easily digestible carbohydrates and proteins. Choose foods like lean meats, white rice, and well-cooked vegetables, which are easier on the digestive system. Avoid high-fat foods such as fried items and fatty cuts of meat, as these can exacerbate symptoms like diarrhea and abdominal pain. Opt for small, frequent meals to aid digestion and reduce discomfort.

Incorporate pancreatic enzyme supplements with each meal to help break down nutrients more efficiently. These supplements can help reduce symptoms like bloating and gas by assisting the digestive process. Always follow the dosage recommendations provided by a healthcare professional, and monitor how different foods affect your symptoms to tailor your diet accordingly.

## Addressing Common EPI Challenges

One common challenge in managing EPI is ensuring adequate nutrient absorption despite reduced pancreatic enzyme activity. To address this, focus on nutrient-dense foods that are easy to digest and consider supplementing with vitamins and minerals if deficiencies are identified. Regular consultations with a dietitian can help adjust your diet and supplements to meet your nutritional needs effectively.

Another challenge is managing digestive discomfort such as gas and bloating. To mitigate these issues, try incorporating probiotic-rich foods like yogurt or kefir into your diet, as they can support gut health and improve digestion. Additionally, avoiding foods that are known to irritate, such as those high in sugar or artificial additives, can help reduce these symptoms.

## Navigating Food Sensitivities and Allergies

When dealing with EPI, it's essential to identify and avoid foods that trigger sensitivities or allergies. Start by keeping a food diary to track what you eat and any symptoms that arise, which can help pinpoint problematic foods. Common allergens like dairy or gluten may need to be excluded if they exacerbate digestive issues, so consider alternatives like lactose-free milk or gluten-free grains.

Substitute problematic ingredients with gut-friendly options to maintain a balanced diet. For example, use almond milk instead of cow's milk if you have lactose intolerance, or choose quinoa instead of wheat if you have gluten sensitivity. Always check ingredient labels carefully to avoid hidden allergens and consult with an allergist or dietitian for personalized advice.

## Practical Tips for Meal Planning and Preparation

Meal planning for EPI involves selecting foods that are both nutritious and easy to digest. Plan your meals around lean proteins, low-fat carbohydrates, and well-cooked vegetables. Preparing meals in advance can save time and ensure you have suitable options available. Batch cooking and freezing portions can help maintain consistency and avoid the temptation of less suitable foods.

Use simple cooking methods such as baking, steaming, or grilling to keep meals light and easy on the digestive system. Avoid heavy sauces or frying, which can add unwanted fat. Keep a list of approved recipes and rotate them to prevent meal fatigue and ensure a varied diet. Utilize kitchen gadgets like slow cookers or food processors to streamline preparation and make meals more convenient.

## Frequently Asked Questions and Expert Advice

**Q: How can I tell if my current diet is managing my EPI effectively?**

Monitor your symptoms and note any changes in digestion or comfort levels. If you experience persistent issues, consult your healthcare provider to adjust your diet or enzyme supplements accordingly. Regular follow-ups can help fine-tune your dietary plan for better symptom control.

**Q: What should I do if I suspect a new food is causing symptoms?**

Eliminate the suspected food from your diet for a period and observe if your symptoms improve. Reintroduce it gradually to confirm if it is the cause. Keeping a detailed food and symptom journal can be valuable in identifying and managing problematic foods.

# 21 Days Meal Plan Recipes plus Ingredients and their Preparations

## DAY 1: Grilled Lemon-Herb Chicken with Quinoa Salad

**Ingredients:**

- 1 boneless, skinless chicken breast
- 2 tbsp olive oil
- Juice of 1 lemon
- 1 tsp dried oregano
- 1 cup quinoa, rinsed
- 2 cups water or low-sodium chicken broth
- 1 cucumber, diced
- 1 tomato, diced
- ¼ cup fresh parsley, chopped
- Salt and pepper to taste

**Preparation:**

- Marinate the chicken with olive oil, lemon juice, oregano, salt, and pepper. Let it sit for 30 minutes.
- Grill chicken over medium heat for 6-8 minutes per side until fully cooked.

- In a pot, bring quinoa and water/broth to a boil. Reduce heat and simmer for 15 minutes until fluffy.

- Mix quinoa with cucumber, tomato, parsley, and additional lemon juice.
- Serve the grilled chicken over the quinoa salad.

## DAY 2: Baked Cod with Steamed Vegetables

**Ingredients:**

- 1 cod fillet
- 1 tbsp olive oil
- Juice of 1 lemon
- 1 tsp dried thyme
- 1 cup broccoli florets
- 1 cup carrots, sliced
- Salt and pepper to taste

**Preparation:**

- Preheat the oven to 375°F (190°C).

- Drizzle cod fillet with olive oil, lemon juice, thyme, salt, and pepper.
- Bake the cod for 12-15 minutes, or until cooked through.
- Steam broccoli and carrots for 5-7 minutes until tender.
- Serve the baked cod with the steamed vegetables on the side.

## DAY 3: Turkey and Zucchini Meatballs with Cauliflower Rice

**Ingredients:**

- 1 lb ground turkey

- 1 zucchini, grated
- 1 egg
- ¼ cup almond flour
- 1 tsp garlic powder
- 1 tsp onion powder
- 1 head cauliflower, grated into rice-size pieces
- 1 tbsp olive oil
- Salt and pepper to taste

**Preparation:**

- Preheat the oven to 400°F (200°C).

- Mix turkey, grated zucchini, egg, almond flour, garlic powder, onion powder, salt, and pepper. Form into meatballs.
- Bake meatballs for 20-25 minutes until golden.
- Sauté cauliflower rice in olive oil for 5 minutes.
- Serve meatballs over cauliflower rice.

## DAY 4: Lemon-Dill Salmon with Asparagus

**Ingredients:**

- 1 salmon fillet
- Juice of 1 lemon
- 1 tsp dried dill
- 1 tbsp olive oil
- 1 bunch of asparagus
- Salt and pepper to taste

**Preparation:**

- Preheat oven to 375°F (190°C).

- Place salmon on a baking sheet and drizzle with olive oil, lemon juice, dill, salt, and pepper.
- Bake salmon for 15-18 minutes until fully cooked.
- Toss asparagus with olive oil, salt, and pepper. Roast alongside salmon for 10-12 minutes.
- Serve salmon with roasted asparagus.

## DAY 5: Chicken Stir-Fry with Zucchini Noodles

**Ingredients:**

- 1 boneless, skinless chicken breast, sliced
- 1 tbsp olive oil
- 1 zucchini, spiralized into noodles
- 1 bell pepper, sliced
- ½ onion, sliced
- 1 tbsp low-sodium soy sauce or tamari
- 1 tsp sesame oil
- 1 tsp garlic powder
- Salt and pepper to taste

**Preparation:**

- Heat olive oil in a skillet and cook chicken until golden brown.
- Add bell pepper and onion, sauté for 5 minutes.
- Stir in zucchini noodles and cook for 2-3 minutes.
- Add soy sauce, sesame oil, garlic powder, salt, and pepper. Stir until well combined.
- Serve warm.

## DAY 6: Herb-crusted chicken with Mashed Sweet Potatoes

**Ingredients:**

- 1 boneless, skinless chicken breast
- 1 tsp dried rosemary
- 1 tsp dried thyme
- 1 tbsp olive oil
- 1 sweet potato, peeled and cubed
- 1 tbsp coconut oil or butter
- Salt and pepper to taste

**Preparation:**

- Preheat oven to 375°F (190°C).
- Rub chicken with rosemary, thyme, olive oil,

salt, and pepper. Bake for 20-25 minutes.

- Boil sweet potatoes for 10-12 minutes until tender.

Drain and mash with coconut oil or butter.

- Serve chicken with mashed sweet potatoes.

## DAY 7: Shrimp and Vegetable Skewers

**Ingredients:**

- 1 cup shrimp, peeled and deveined
- 1 zucchini, sliced
- 1 bell pepper, chopped
- ½ onion, chopped
- 1 tbsp olive oil
- Juice of 1 lime
- 1 tsp garlic powder
- Salt and pepper to taste

**Preparation:**

- Preheat the grill to medium heat.
- Thread shrimp, zucchini, bell pepper, and onion onto skewers.
- Drizzle with olive oil, lime juice, garlic powder, salt, and pepper.
- Grill for 3-4 minutes per side until shrimp is cooked through.
- Serve warm.

## DAY 8: Grilled Chicken with Roasted Brussels Sprouts

**Ingredients:**

- 1 boneless, skinless chicken breast

- 1 tbsp olive oil
- Juice of 1 lemon
- 1 tsp paprika
- 1 cup Brussels sprouts, halved
- Salt and pepper to taste

**Preparation:**

- Marinate chicken with olive oil, lemon juice,

paprika, salt, and pepper for 30 minutes.

- Grill chicken for 6-8 minutes per side until fully cooked.
- Toss Brussels sprouts with olive oil, salt, and pepper. Roast at 400°F (200°C) for 20-25 minutes.
- Serve the grilled chicken with roasted Brussels sprouts.

## DAY 9: Baked Tilapia with Spinach

**Ingredients:**

- 1 tilapia fillet
- 1 tbsp olive oil
- Juice of 1 lemon
- 1 tsp dried basil
- 2 cups fresh spinach
- Salt and pepper to taste

**Preparation:**

- Preheat oven to 375°F (190°C).

- Place tilapia on a baking sheet and drizzle with olive oil, lemon juice, basil, salt, and pepper.
- Bake for 10-12 minutes until fully cooked.
- Sauté spinach in a pan with olive oil for 2-3 minutes until wilted.
- Serve the tilapia with sautéed spinach.

## DAY 10: Turkey and Vegetable Skillet

**Ingredients:**

- 1 cup ground turkey
- 1 tbsp olive oil
- 1 zucchini, chopped
- 1 bell pepper, chopped
- ½ onion, chopped
- 1 tsp garlic powder
- Salt and pepper to taste

**Preparation:**

- Heat olive oil in a skillet. Cook ground turkey until browned.
- Add zucchini, bell pepper, and onion. Sauté for 5-7 minutes.
- Season with garlic powder, salt, and pepper.
- Serve warm.

## DAY 11: Lemon-garlic shrimp with Steamed Broccoli

**Ingredients:**

- 1 cup shrimp, peeled and deveined
- 1 tbsp olive oil
- Juice of 1 lemon
- 1 garlic clove, minced
- 1 cup broccoli florets
- Salt and pepper to taste

**Preparation:**

- Heat olive oil in a pan and sauté garlic for 1 minute.
- Add shrimp and cook for 3-4 minutes per side.
- Drizzle with lemon juice, salt, and pepper.
- Steam broccoli for 5-7 minutes until tender.
- Serve shrimp with steamed broccoli.

## DAY 12: Chicken and Broccoli Stir-Fry

**Ingredients:**

- 1 boneless, skinless chicken breast, sliced
- 1 tbsp olive oil
- 1 cup broccoli florets
- ½ onion, sliced
- 1 tbsp low-sodium soy sauce
- 1 tsp garlic powder
- Salt and pepper to taste

**Preparation:**

- Heat olive oil in a skillet and cook chicken until golden brown.
- Add broccoli and onion. Sauté for 5-7 minutes.
- Stir in soy sauce, garlic powder, salt, and pepper.
- Serve warm.

## DAY 13: Grilled Salmon with Quinoa and Roasted Vegetables

**Ingredients:**

- 1 salmon fillet
- 1 tbsp olive oil
- Juice of 1 lemon
- 1 tsp dried dill
- 1 cup quinoa, rinsed
- 2 cups water or chicken broth
- 1 cup mixed vegetables (zucchini, bell pepper, carrots)
- Salt and pepper to taste

**Preparation:**

- Preheat the grill to medium heat.
- Marinate salmon with olive oil, lemon juice, dill, salt, and pepper. Grill for 15-18 minutes.
- In a pot, bring quinoa and water/broth to a boil. Reduce heat and simmer for 15 minutes.
- Roast mixed vegetables with olive oil, salt, and pepper at 400°F (200°C) for 20 minutes.

- Serve grilled salmon with quinoa and roasted vegetables.

## DAY 14: Herb-Roasted Chicken with Sweet Potato Wedges

**Ingredients:**

- 1 boneless, skinless chicken breast
- 1 tbsp olive oil
- 1 tsp dried rosemary
- 1 tsp dried thyme
- 1 sweet potato, cut into wedges
- Salt and pepper to taste

**Preparation:**

- Preheat oven to 375°F (190°C).
- Rub chicken with olive oil, rosemary, thyme, salt, and pepper.
- Roast chicken for 20-25 minutes.
- Toss sweet potato wedges with olive oil, salt, and pepper. Roast for 25-30 minutes.

Serve the roasted chicken with sweet potato wedges.

## DAY 15: Turkey Stuffed Bell Peppers

- **Ingredients:**
- 4 bell peppers (any color)
- 1 cup ground turkey
- 1 cup cooked quinoa
- 1 cup diced tomatoes
- 1 tsp dried basil
- 1 tsp dried oregano
- 1 tbsp olive oil
- Salt and pepper to taste
- **Preparation:**
- Preheat oven to 375°F (190°C).

- Cut tops off bell peppers and remove seeds.
- In a skillet, heat olive oil and cook ground turkey until browned.
- Mix in quinoa, diced tomatoes, basil, oregano, salt, and pepper.
- Stuff the bell peppers with the turkey mixture. Place in a baking dish and cover with foil.
- Bake for 30 minutes, then remove foil and bake for an additional 10 minutes.
- Serve warm.

## DAY 16: Lemon Garlic Tilapia with Steamed Green Beans

**Ingredients:**

- 1 tilapia fillet
- 1 tbsp olive oil
- Juice of 1 lemon
- 1 garlic clove, minced
- 1 cup green beans
- Salt and pepper to taste

**Preparation:**

- Preheat oven to 375°F (190°C).
- Place tilapia on a baking sheet and drizzle with olive oil, lemon juice, garlic, salt, and pepper.
- Bake for 10-12 minutes until tilapia is cooked through.
- Steam green beans for 5-7 minutes until tender.
- Serve tilapia with steamed green beans.

## DAY 17: Chicken and Sweet Potato Hash

**Ingredients:**

- 1 boneless, skinless chicken breast, diced
- 1 sweet potato, peeled and diced
- 1 red bell pepper, diced
- ½ onion, diced
- 1 tbsp olive oil
- 1 tsp smoked paprika

Salt and pepper to taste

**Preparation:**

- Heat olive oil in a skillet. Cook chicken until browned and cooked through. Remove from skillet.
- Add sweet potato, bell pepper, and onion to the same skillet. Cook until the sweet potato is tender.
- Return chicken to the skillet, add paprika, salt, and pepper. Mix well and cook for an additional 2-3 minutes.
- Serve warm.

## DAY 18: Baked Chicken Thighs with Steamed Broccoli

**Ingredients:**

- 2 chicken thighs, bone-in, skinless
- 1 tbsp olive oil
- 1 tsp dried rosemary
- 1 tsp dried thyme
- 1 cup broccoli florets
- Salt and pepper to taste

**Preparation:**

- Preheat oven to 375°F (190°C).
- Rub chicken thighs with olive oil, rosemary, thyme, salt, and pepper.
- Bake for 30-35 minutes until fully cooked.
- Steam broccoli for 5-7 minutes until tender.
- Serve chicken thighs with steamed broccoli.

## DAY 19: Turkey and Spinach Stuffed Mushrooms

**Ingredients:**

- 6 large mushrooms, stems removed
- 1 cup ground turkey
- 1 cup fresh spinach, chopped
- 1 garlic clove, minced
- 1 tbsp olive oil
- ¼ cup almond flour
- Salt and pepper to taste

**Preparation:**

- Preheat oven to 375°F (190°C).
- In a skillet, heat olive oil and cook ground turkey until browned.
- Add spinach and garlic to the skillet and cook until spinach is wilted.
- Stir in almond flour, salt, and pepper.
- Stuff mushroom caps with the turkey mixture.
- Place stuffed mushrooms in a baking dish and bake for 15-20 minutes.
- Serve warm.

## DAY 20: Grilled Shrimp and Avocado Salad

**Ingredients:**

- 1 cup shrimp, peeled and deveined
- 1 tbsp olive oil
- Juice of 1 lime
- 1 avocado, diced
- 2 cups mixed salad greens
- 1 cucumber, sliced
- 1 tbsp fresh cilantro, chopped
- Salt and pepper to taste

**Preparation:**

- Preheat the grill to medium heat.

- Toss shrimp with olive oil, lime juice, salt, and pepper. Grill for 3-4 minutes per side.

- Toss salad greens, cucumber, avocado, and cilantro in a bowl.
- Top salad with grilled shrimp.
- Serve immediately.

## DAY 21: Lemon-Basil Chicken with Roasted Carrots

**Ingredients:**

- 1 boneless, skinless chicken breast
- 1 tbsp olive oil
- Juice of 1 lemon
- 1 tsp dried basil
- 1 cup carrots, sliced
- Salt and pepper to taste

**Preparation:**

- Preheat oven to 375°F (190°C).
- Rub chicken breast with olive oil, lemon juice, basil, salt, and pepper.

- Bake chicken for 20-25 minutes until cooked through.
- Toss carrots with olive oil, salt, and pepper. Roast for 20-25 minutes.
- Serve chicken with roasted carrots.
- This completes your 21-day meal plan, offering a variety of recipes that are both gut-friendly and supportive of pancreatic health.

## Author's appreciation

Thank you for embarking on this culinary journey with me through "Easy, Gut-Friendly Recipes for Managing EPI Symptoms, Boosting Digestion, and Supporting Pancreatic Health." Your commitment to improving your well-being through thoughtful dietary choices is truly commendable.

I hope these recipes provide not only relief from the symptoms of Exocrine Pancreatic Insufficiency (EPI) but also inspire you to explore new flavors and embrace a healthier lifestyle.

Each meal has been crafted with care to ensure that it supports your digestive health while delighting your taste buds.

Remember, managing EPI is a journey, and every small step you take toward better nutrition is a victory. May these recipes bring you comfort, satisfaction, and improved health.

Thank you for trusting me to be a part of your wellness journey. Wishing you health, happiness, and many delicious meals ahead by following this meal plan

Made in the USA
Las Vegas, NV
24 October 2024